The Funny Side Collection
The Fart Side
Bottoms Up!
(Expanded Full Blast Edition!)

Dan Reynolds
Joseph Weiss, MD

© 2017 Dan Reynolds
　　　　Joseph Weiss, M.D.
　　　　SmartAsk Books
　　　　Rancho Santa Fe, California, USA
　　　　www.smartaskbooks.com

All rights reserved. No part of this book may be reproduced, reused, republished, or retransmitted in any form, or stored in a database or retrieval system, without written permission of the publisher.

ISBN-13: 978-1-943760-57-2 (Color Print Expanded)
ISBN-13: 978-1-943760-62-6 (e-Book Expanded)
ISBN-13: 978-1-943760-50-3 (Color Print Pocket Rocket)
ISBN-13: 978-1-943760-51-0 (e-Book Pocket Rocket)

The Fart Side: Bottoms Up!

Methane is not produced by bacteria, but by other microbes known as Archaea.

The flammability of intestinal gas results when methane and/or hydrogen are produced. If the ignited gas has a blue flame it signifies that methane is present. The lighting of intestinal gas is not without risk and can lead to injury.

Because humans continue to regress even as technology progresses, there are at least 60 apps for smart phones which recreate the sound of human flatulence.

Other gases that contribute to the characteristic fecal odor include indole, skatole, ammonia, and mercaptans. They commonly arise with the digestion of tryptophan, animal proteins and fats.

The Fart Side: Bottoms Up!

The Ontario Ministry of Health embarked on a public education campaign to curb tobacco usage. A common theme used by smokers to avoid the stigma of nicotine addiction was to describe their habit as a social smoker. The public education campaign focused on the denial as being analogous to describing oneself as a social farter, that is a person who enjoyed farting while in the company of others.

If the average person farts fourteen times a day, by eighty years of age they will have farted about 41,000 times.

Pythagoras of Samos (c.570 BCE - c.495 BCE) was a Greek philosopher and mathematician. Pythagoras demanded that his adherents abstain from eating beans to avoid flatulence, as he believed that with every fart a small portion of the soul escaped.

The Fart Side: Bottoms Up!

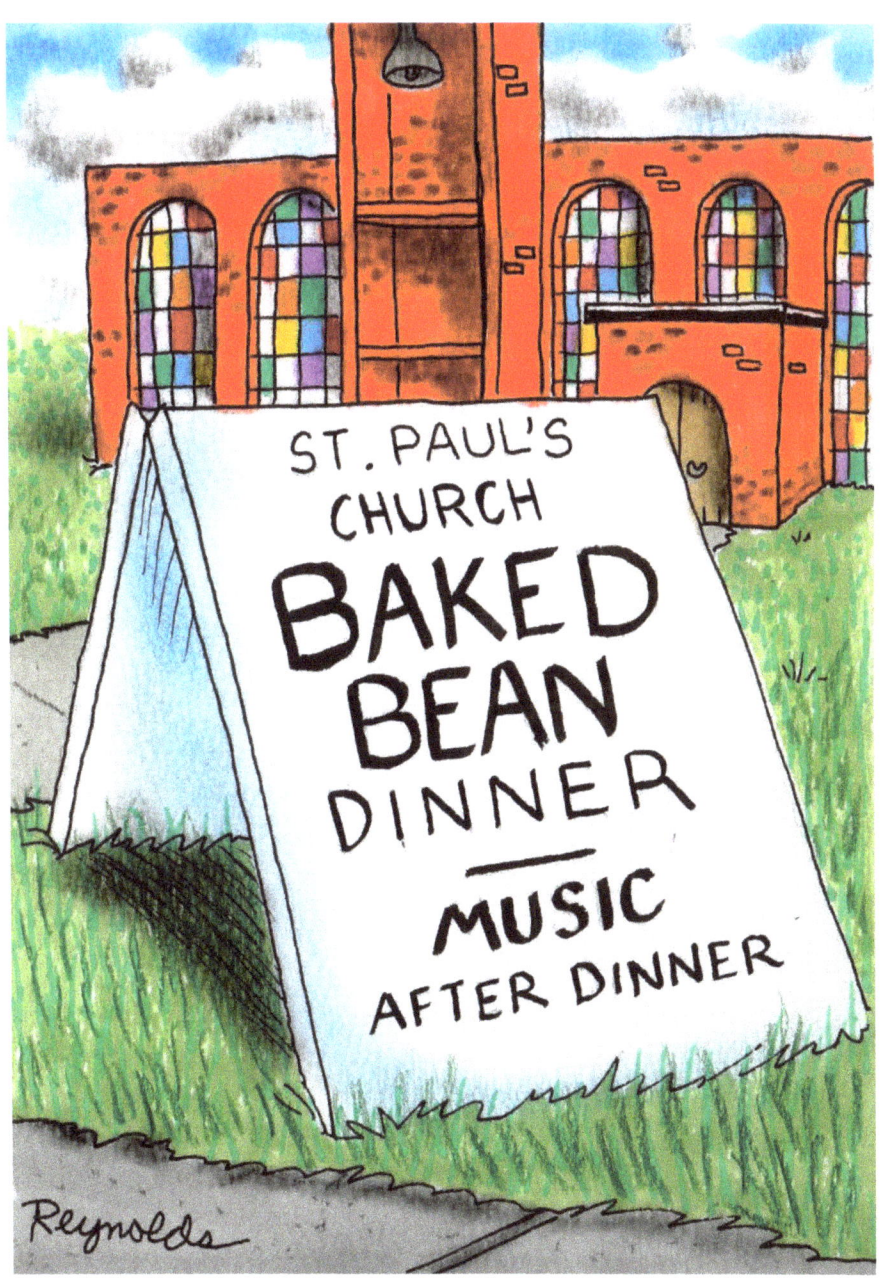

Inhaling some farts may be healthy. According to researchers at Exeter University, sniffing tiny amounts of hydrogen sulfide can reverse mitochondrial damage and help avert strokes, dementia, cancer, and heart attacks.

"Professional Fart Smeller" is a job in China. These talented professionals make up to $50,000 a year by diagnosing digestive illnesses, merely through the scent of the patient's flatulence.

Some beetles fart to attract mates. The female Southern Pine Beetle releases sex attractant hormones, known as pheromones, in their farts to attract male suitors.

Digestive diseases are one of the most prevalent causes of disability in the work force.

The Fart Side: Bottoms Up!

There is a marine creature that farts into its mouth. Crinoid, also known as the "Sea Lily", has an intestinal tract that is U-shaped, which means that its flatulence is released adjacent to its own mouth.

Half of all women admit that they have farted during sex. According to a study at the University of California San Francisco 43% of women surveyed reported that they'd experienced 'flatus incontinence' with sex over the previous three months. Males refused to admit that they farted during sex.

Elagabalus, a Roman Emperor who was assassinated at age eighteen, was known for using whoopee cushions as a practical joke.

The gastrointestinal tract is twenty-three feet long, about the vertical height of a two-story building.

The Fart Side: Bottoms Up!

"Mr. McCarthy, you have a condition known as Explosive Ass Syndrome."

According to tradition, Germans considered it impolite if their guests did not burp. It's a way of telling the host that you are satisfied with the meal just consumed.

German religious reformer Martin Luther used to say, "*Warum pfurzet und ruelpset ihr nicht, hat es euch nicht geschmecket?*" which translates to, "*Why don't you farteth and burpeth? Didn't you fancy the meal?*"

Women release greater quantities of the gas hydrogen sulfide, which has a foul rotten egg smell, in their farts than men.

The name mammal is derived from mammary glands, the medical term for the breasts which produce milk.

Digestive diseases account for twenty-five percent of all surgical operations.

The Fart Side: Bottoms Up!

Aristotle (384 BC–322 BCE) was a prominent Greek philosopher and polymath. He was a student of Plato, and the teacher and friend of Alexander the Great. Aristotle wrote on the digestive problems of elephants with flatulence in his work *Historia Animalium*.

Nearly thirty thousand trees a day are converted into toilet paper.

It can take your gut flora up to a year to fully repopulate itself after just one course of antibiotics.

Cicero's famous Farticus was possibly the world's first limerick:
There once was a man named Farticus
Who bravely fought beside Spartacus.
He let one rip,
His gladius slipped,
And we smelled no more of this Farticus.

The Fart Side: Bottoms Up!

Even though they are dairy products, hard cheeses and yogurt often have relatively low lactose content.

A high fat meal slows down gut motility and transport, allowing more microbial fermentation, which results in the greater production of intestinal gas.

Although most farts are invisible under ordinary circumstances, it is not difficult to make them readily visible by farting underwater.

Hydrogen sulfide is a poisonous gas with a rotten egg smell that the human nose can detect at very low concentrations. When the gas concentration is high, the nose cannot detect it at all.

The gallbladder is not a vital organ for digestion.

The Fart Side: Bottoms Up!

Farting is more likely to occur in elevators while they are going up in high rise buildings, than in those exact same elevators going down.

The potency and aroma of the farts of boys increases as they go through puberty and reach adulthood.

Females have a heightened sense of smell at the time of ovulation during the menstrual cycle.

William Shakespeare refers to a fart in one of his plays.

US President Lyndon Johnson insulted future US President Gerald Ford by claiming he wasn't smart enough to chew gum and fart at the same time.

The stomach hydrochloric acid can dissolve metal, and burn skin on contact, but it cannot dissolve plastic.

The Fart Side: Bottoms Up!

Her toes in the sand. The wind at his back. They were living the dream.

Roman Emperor Claudius decreed that citizens of Rome could fart in public. He believed that holding back a fart could lead to illness or death.

Wolfgang Amadeus Mozart was fascinated and obsessed with farts and scatological matter.

Richard Wagner often complained about his bowel problems, and described his farts by the musical notes and keys they played.

Joseph Pujol, known by the name Le Pétomane (The Farter in French) was the highest paid stage performer of his day, playing Le Marseilles by farting out the tune on the Moulin Rouge in Paris.

The neurotransmitter serotonin is found in much higher concentrations in the gut, than in the brain.

The Fart Side: Bottoms Up!

Prominent fart scenes have occurred in hundreds of Hollywood movies, including Walt Disney films for children.

The famous Greek mathematician Pythagoras believed that beans should not be consumed because a small portion of the soul escaped with each fart. He was so opposed to harming bean plants that he refused to flee across a bean field to escape from the assassins who killed him.

Over four billion people around the world never use toilet paper.

The average speed of a fart is indirectly measured by the diffusion of its smell, which has been recorded as greater than ten miles per hour.

There are over one thousand six hundred known digestive enzymes.

The Fart Side: Bottoms Up!

Morticians secure the anus of the deceased closed so that an audible fart does not frighten attendees at a memorial service or funeral.

Farting has become more accepted in Western society, with frequent references to it and the treatments available, in the media.

Using toilet paper is not hygienic, as the paper is thin and porous. Toilet paper is an inferior form of anal hygiene compared to water from a bidet.

The pastry delicacy Pets de Nonne, which means 'Nun's Farts' in French, is named such because they are heavenly light and airy.

Certain insects can walk on water because of the physical property of surface tension.

The Fart Side: Bottoms Up!

Pumpernickel is the German word for 'Devil's Farts', and the coarse grain of the bread often leads to pungent farting.

The farts of carnivores smell more offensive than the farts of vegetarians.

About thirty percent of people produce flammable farts.

The flammable gasses that may be found in a fart include oxygen, hydrogen, and methane.

Most people lose the lactase enzyme to digest the milk sugar lactose shortly after weaning. Lactose intolerance may exhibit symptoms that can include excess gas and cramps.

Methane has a characteristic blue flame. If your farts burn with a blue flame, you are a methane producer.

The Fart Side: Bottoms Up!

Despite their efforts to be credible, the pro-dad group did nothing but raise a stink.

Metrocles (c.325 BCE), a philosopher who studied in Aristotle's Lyceum, accidentally farted in public while practicing a speech. He was so embarrassed that he attempted to commit suicide by starvation.

The average person goes to the toilet two thousand five-hundred times per year, and spends a total of three years of their lifetime sitting on the toilet.

Tiberius Claudius Caesar Augustus Germanicus (13 BCE – 54 AD), commonly known as Claudius, became the fourth emperor of the Roman Empire upon the assassination of his predecessor Caligula. Claudius had been made aware of an individual who had died as the result of a retained fart. To protect his citizens from a similar ill wind of fate, he decreed that all citizens of Rome could fart at will in public or in private.

The Fart Side: Bottoms Up!

Mom, Dad said he was bitten by a radioactive stink bug which gave him a superpower. What is it?

An apple is forty percent air by volume, and increases intestinal gas.

Meteorism is an old English term for farting.

Women and girls fart with the same frequency as men, but in smaller volumes.

Poor fitting dentures can contribute to intestinal gas by air swallowing, known as aerophagia.

Drinking from a straw, bottle, or can may lead to an increase in air swallowing and intestinal gas.

Chewing gum, tobacco, or ruminating can lead to increased aerophagia and intestinal gas.

Over four billion people around the world never use toilet paper.

The Fart Side: Bottoms Up!

"Your baked beans are out of this world, honey... honey???"

About thirty percent of the human population are methane producers, which contributes to global warming. They produce flammable farts.

Scuba divers are advised to avoid beans before a dive because of the expanding gas issue on ascent.

Aristophanes (c. 446 BCE – c. 386 BCE) was a comical playwright of Ancient Greece. His 5th century BC plays The Knights and The Clouds, contain numerous fart jokes. *The Clouds*:" First, think of a tiny fart that your intestines make. Then consider the heavens: their infinite farting is thunder. For thunder and farting are, in principle, one and the same.

In the U.S., more than fifty miles (eighty kilometers) of toilet paper is produced every second of the day and night throughout the year.

The Fart Side: Bottoms Up!

The ten liters of air swallowed every day by the average person is seventy-eight percent nitrogen. Nitrogen is not well absorbed by the intestinal tract, and must be released as either a burp or as a fart.

Most people burp and fart while they sleep, and occasionally it is loud or aromatic enough to wake themselves or a sleeping partner.

Beer poured in the mile-high city of Denver will have a larger head of bubbles than the same beer poured in Seattle. The difference is due to atmospheric pressure and altitude.

Gelato compared to ice cream has a lower calorie content by weight, but a higher calorie content by volume.

Nearly thirty thousand trees a day are converted into toilet paper.

The Fart Side: Bottoms Up!

The largest organ or tissue of the body exposed to the external environment is the gastrointestinal tract. The inside lumen of the gut is considered external to the body.

Thomas Moore (1478 – 1535) was a philosopher, statesmen, humanist, and theologian, who was canonized to sainthood by the Pope. King Henry VIII beheaded him when he refused to accept papal authority regarding his marriage to Catherine of Aragon. In 1518, Sir Thomas More, in an epigram entitled *In Efflatum Ventis*, wrote "'Wind, if you keep it too long in your stomach, kills you; on the other hand, it can save your life if it is properly let out. If wind can save or destroy you, then is it not as powerful as dreaded kings?'"

Worldwide two million people die each year from diarrhea.

The Fart Side: Bottoms Up!

Living at high altitude, such as Denver or Mexico City, significantly increases intestinal gas volume, because of lower atmospheric pressure.

Anal scent glands are often used as territorial markers in the animal world. They are one reason dogs frequently smell each other's droppings to identify their scent.

Going up in an elevator in a high-rise building increases farting, because intestinal gasses expand as the atmospheric pressure decreases.

The US Department of Agriculture has supported research to develop a bean with lower concentrations of the sugars that lead to flatulence.

Toilet seats in most U.S. homes have lower microbial populations than kitchen faucets and handles.

The Fart Side: Bottoms Up!

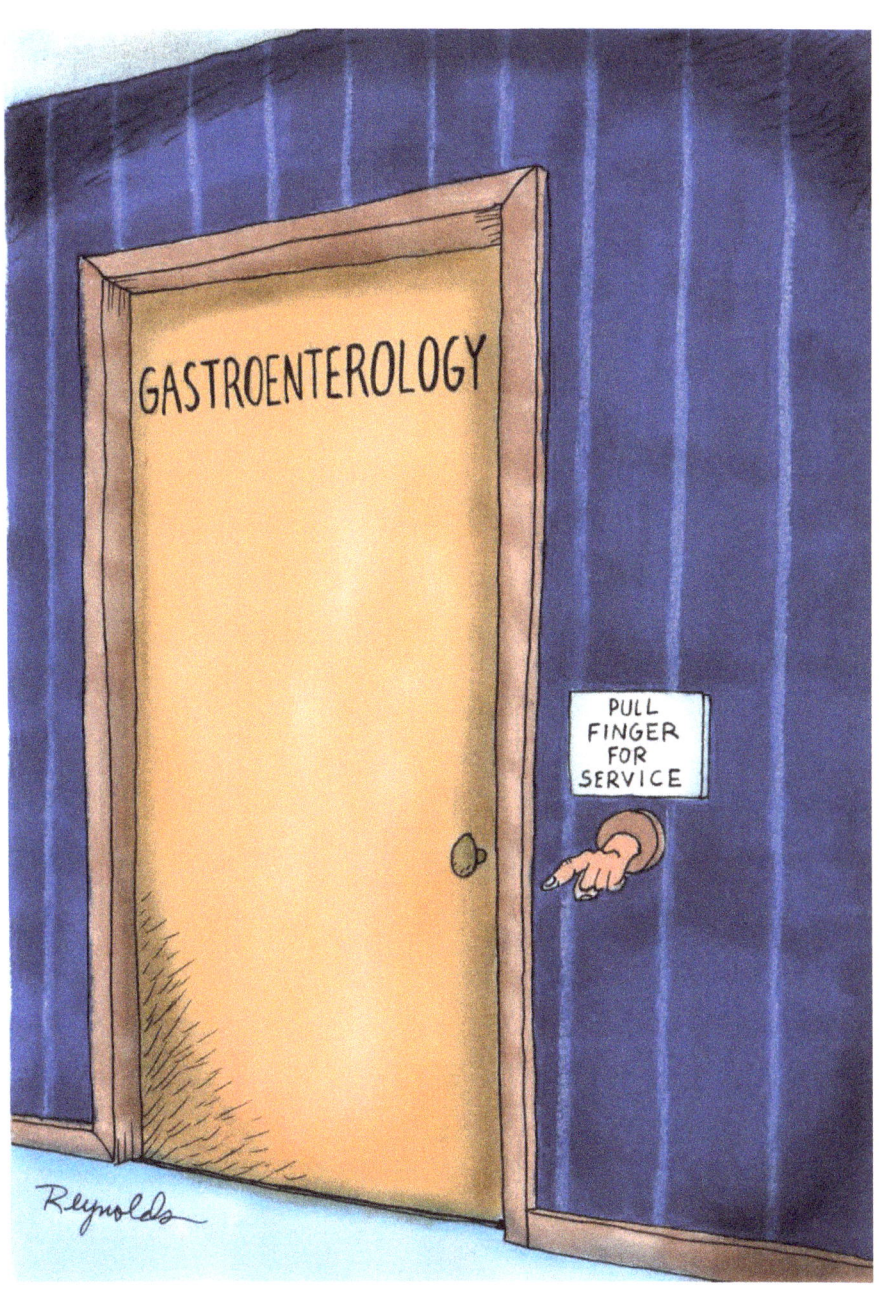

Although about thirty percent of people enjoy the aroma of their own farts, a smaller percentage enjoys the aroma of the farts of others.

The psychiatric condition of deriving sexual pleasure and gratification from farts is known as eproctophilia.

Adolf Hitler had extreme flatulence. He was prescribed anti-gas pills that contained arsenic, and may have contributed to his mental illness.

If the average person parts fourteen times a day, by eighty years of age they will have farted about 41,000 times.

Burping after a meal is a compliment to the hostess in several Asian cultures.

In ten years, a mattress will double in weight with dust mites and their feces.

The Fart Side: Bottoms Up!

How fast does a fart travel? About ten feet per second, which works out to about seven miles per hour. It would take a fart a little more than three hours to run a standard marathon.

The average speed of a fart leaving the anus is about ten feet per second or about 9.5 km/hr.

Gerald Ford, 38th U.S. President would blame his farts on the Secret Service by loudly proclaiming, "Jesus, was that you? Show some class!"

Carbon Dioxide gas is easily absorbed by the gut, enters into solution in the blood, and is eliminated from the body by being exhaled via the lungs.

There are on average one hundred times more bacterial contaminants on restaurant menus than on restaurant toilet seats.

The Fart Side: Bottoms Up!

The sensory nerves within your rectum can tell the difference between a fart and poop. They can distinguish between the different sensations of solid, liquid, and gas. The only exception is with diarrhea when the liquid stool can be released with the passage of gas, commonly described as a shart.

Two thirds of adults pass farts that contain no methane. If both parents are methane producers, their children have a ninety-five percent chance of being producers as well. Since methane producers are an elite group (only one third of the population), a special club called the Royal Order of the Blue Flame has been established just for that them. Methane burns with a characteristic blue flame.

Thirty thousand trees a day are harvested and made into toilet paper.

The Fart Side: Bottoms Up!

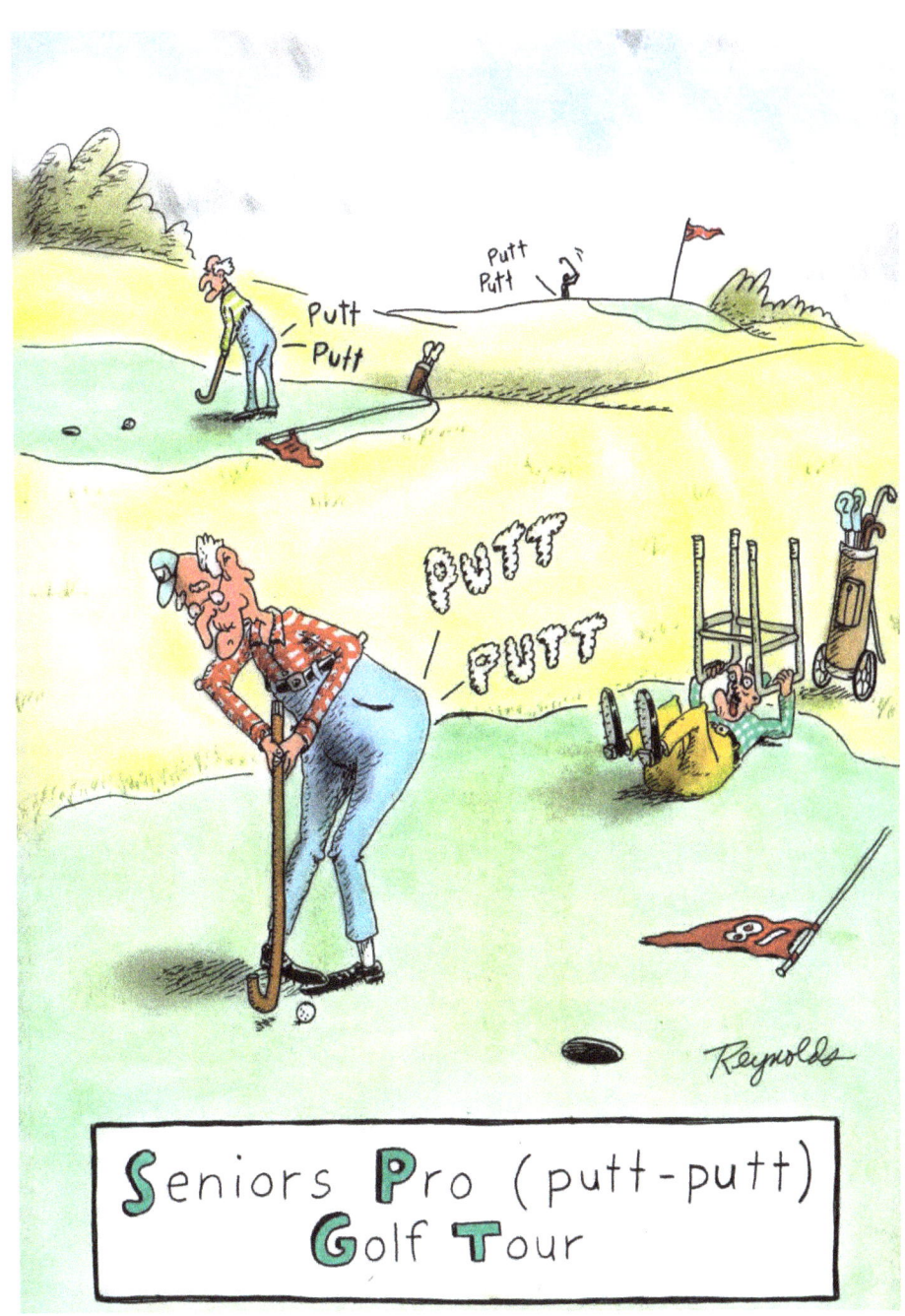

Marcus Tullius Cicero (106 BCE – 43 BCE) was a Roman philosopher, statesman, lawyer, and orator. Cicero wrote: "The fart as well as the burp must be permitted. Cicero's *Heuristics* starts with "Open with a fart joke, use Farticus if you don't have another."

Desiderius Erasmus Roterodamus (1466–1536) was a Dutch Renaissance humanist, classical scholar, social, and theologian who was an advocate for religious toleration. His comments on farting include: "Do not move back and forth on your chair. Doing so gives the impression of constantly breaking, or trying to break, wind. Retain the wind by compressing the belly."

In the U.S., more than fifty miles (eighty kilometers) of toilet paper is produced every second of the day and night, throughout the year.

The Fart Side: Bottoms Up!

Traveling to higher altitudes, such as mountain climbing, airplane travel, hot air balloon, etc. results in exposure to reduced atmospheric pressure, which causes intestinal gasses to expand.

Dogs and cats are carnivores with a protein-rich diet which produces relatively small amounts of intestinal gas, but with a pungent aroma. The dietary proteins often contain sulfur. A dog's or cat's farts are not often heard, but the odor is potent.

Large herbivorous animals such as cows, horses, and elephants, produce vast quantities of intestinal gas. The aroma is not as offensive as meat eaters because of the lack of sulfur in the protein of their vegetarian diet.

More than twenty-five billion rolls of toilet paper are sold every year in the U.S.

The Fart Side: Bottoms Up!

Fish have an air bladder, which is independent of the gastrointestinal tract. It serves to control buoyancy.

Fish, like all living creatures, generate gas within their intestinal tract which is released as a fart. It has an unexplored role in fish buoyancy, but does not rival the air bladder in this important function.

Reptiles including turtles and snakes fart, with sound and smell. The Sonoran coral snake and hook-nosed snake fart with an audible popping sound when disturbed.

The fart bubble of a blue whale is so large when it reaches the surface of the ocean that it can envelope a horse and rider, and asphyxiate them both.

Sipping smaller volumes increases the amount of air swallowed (aerophagia).

The Fart Side: Bottoms Up!

As a fart is defined as an anal escape of intestinal gas, animals that lack an intestinal tract or an anus do not fart. An example would be the sponge, which does not have specialized organs.

The cnidarians are an animal phylum that includes the jellyfish, corals, sea anemones and hydra. Their tissues are organized into a digestive pouch with a mouth surrounded by stinging tentacles. Food enters the mouth and is digested inside the pouch, after which the leftovers are expelled via the same opening. In effect, the same opening thus serves as both a mouth and an anus. Any gas expelled by a cnidarian would be more termed a belch rather than a fart, since the animal lacks intestines as well as an anus.

Air is seventy-eight percent nitrogen, which is poorly absorbed by the gut.

The Fart Side: Bottoms Up!

Another group of animals that don't fart are those that live very deep underwater, but nor because they do not have an anus. Living so deep below the sea surface, they are under enormous atmospheric pressure from the heavy volume of water above them. The pressure is so high that the gas remains in solution, rather than forming bubbles. Clams, echinoderms, fish, and other animals living near the deep ocean seafloor do not fart, because their gasses stay in solution and never emerge as bubbles. If they are placed in shallower waters with less atmospheric pressure, they may begin to fart for the very first time!

The explosive release of a high-pressure fart may eject feces at high velocity, much like a cannon ball. When the feces are more liquid, as in cases of diarrhea, the release of a fart with liquid feces is known as a shart.

The Fart Side: Bottoms Up!

In World War Two, the Air Force operated B-17 bombers which were not pressurized. Airmen in rapidly ascending aircraft were exposed to the diminished atmospheric pressure when at a cruising altitude of 20,000 feet above sea level. The lower atmospheric pressure at this altitude caused the pockets of gas in their gastrointestinal tract to expand, causing what was later defined as HAFE (high altitude flatus expulsion). Severe abdominal pain, barotrauma, intestinal rupture, and death were possible complications if they could not release the gas quickly enough.

Farts in the confined space of a shower stall have a stronger olfactory presence, because of the added effects of high humidity and temperature.

Poor fitting dentures can contribute to intestinal gas

The Fart Side: Bottoms Up!

The chemical capsaicin, found in hot chili peppers and other hot spices, causes stimulation of the sensitive temperature nerve receptors. Capsaicin applied to the skin or mucous membranes results in a burning sensation. When ingested, it can pass through the gastrointestinal tract, and cause a burning sensation in the rectum and anus.

A rare condition of a colovaginal fistula, an abnormal passageway between the bowel and the vagina, can lead to the passage of intestinal gas and feces out through the female genitalia. A fistula to the urinary bladder can result in urinary tract infections as well as peumaturia, air bubbles in the urine of men or women.

Sternutation is the formal term for a sneeze.

The Fart Side: Bottoms Up!

Ice cream is often forty percent air by volume, and leads to intestinal gas.

Trapped air in the vagina can be expelled with sexual intercourse or exertion. It is not a true fart, and does not have the characteristic odor of a fart, but it can sound like one. It is often referred to as a queef. In Great Britain, this phenomenon is called a "fanny fart." in Great Britain, the word fanny pertains to the female genitalia. In the U.S 'fanny' refers to the buttocks.

Eructation is the formal term for a belch or burp.

Tussis is the formal term for a cough.

A hiccup is caused by the involuntary contraction of the diaphragm

Mastication is the formal term for chewing

The Fart Side: Bottoms Up!

Although many liters of carbon dioxide gas are produced when stomach acid is neutralized by pancreatic secretions, it is rapidly absorbed and exhaled.

Augustine of Hippo (St. Augustine) (354 AD – 430-AD) was a Christian philosopher and theologian. In his treatise on *City of God* he comments on the passing of intestinal gas. He describes individuals that "have such command of their bowels, that they can break wind continuously at will, so as to produce the effect of singing".

Michel Eyquem de Montaigne (1533-1592) was a French Renaissance author, statesman, physician, essayist, and sufferer of chronic constipation. "God alone knows how many times our bellies, by the refusal of one single fart, have brought us to the door of an agonizing death."

The Fart Side: Bottoms Up!

Farts that pass-through clothing and filtering material, especially if it contains activated charcoal, lose some of their potency. The molecules of odorants, as well as microscopic droplets of feces, become trapped in the clothing fibers.

The streaks and marks on underwear are partly due to lack of total anal hygiene after a bowel movement, as well as the particulate residue of farts carrying microscopic fecal material.

If internal bleeding is occurring in the gastrointestinal tract, especially in the rectum or anus, it is possible to disperse a spray of blood with a vigorous fart. It can also occur in a menstruating female who has a queef.

The average person swallows every thirty seconds while awake, and every five minutes while asleep.

The Fart Side: Bottoms Up!

When one passes a quiet fart, especially a very odiferous type known as a silent but deadly (SBD) fart, the natural inclination is to walk some distance away so as not be identified as the source. This is often a failed maneuver because the contributor's clothing retains a lingering trace, and the walking away creates a flow of turbulence of the aroma. An olfactory trail leading directly to the culprit.

A space suit contains the propulsive force of a fart. Without a spacesuit, its energy would lead the body of the farting astronaut to move in the opposite direction. Its propulsive motion would be heightened because it is unopposed because of the lack of friction in the vacuum of outer space.

External hemorrhoids are often painful, while internal hemorrhoids are always painless.

The Fart Side: Bottoms Up!

Termite farts have been trapped in amber, the petrified sap of trees, for thousands of years. Fossil farts preserved in amber have been analyzed by gas chromatography, confirming that they contain methane gas, just like from present day termites.

Technically, it is not the termites that generate the methane gas but the Archaea microbes that reside in the termite's digestive tract. Archaea ferment the cellulose in the termite diet.

The microbes continued to generate the gasses for some time after the termite died in the amber, allowing the last post-mortem farts of the termite to be trapped as bubbles visible and ready to be analyzed thousands of years later, as their last gift to human knowledge.

The Fart Side: Bottoms Up!

Immanuel Kant (1724 –1804) was a German Prussian philosopher. Kant described hypochondriac winds as farts when raging in the guts, and as heavenly visions when raging in the mind. Kant saw in the farting mystic a parody of himself.

Sir Winston Spencer Churchill (1874-1965) was a British statesmen and Prime Minister during the Second World War. At a dinner party Sir Winston reportedly farted audibly. An offended gentleman reproached him saying "How dare you pass wind in front of my wife!" Sir Winston's quick witted response was "I am sorry; I did not know it was her turn."

The internal anal sphincter relaxes involuntarily when stool is present in the rectum. It is the external anal sphincter under voluntary control that maintains continence.

The Fart Side: Bottoms Up!

Eproctophilia is a fart fetish, the receiving of sexual pleasure and arousal from the fart of another.

Carbon dioxide gas is heavier than air.

Farts are found in classical art history, and are illustrated by the works of Hieronymus Bosch (c. 1450 – 1516). He was a Dutch artist known for his famous triptych *The Garden of Earthly Delights*. It illustrates a nude figure farting roses, and a nude playing the flute from his rear end.

The expression 'the fart of the water goblin' in Japanese means something small and insignificant. If the water goblin does it in the water, it is not heard and does not smell.

There are over one thousand six hundred known digestive enzymes.

The Fart Side: Bottoms Up!

In Japan, several individuals earned a living as performers who could utilize their farts for entertainment.

Pieter Bruegel (Brueghel) the Elder (c. 1525 –1569) was an artist of the Flemish Renaissance famous for the painting *Netherlandish Proverbs* which illustrates several Dutch proverbs and sayings. The proverbs 'It hangs like a privy over a ditch' and 'They both crap and fart through the same hole' are illustrated by a scene of exposed buttocks above a river.

George Cruikshank (1792-1878) was a British caricaturist, illustrator and satirist. In one of his illustrations the Prince of Wales is farting on his own loyal subjects petitioning for reform.

Over four billion people around the world never use toilet paper.

The Fart Side: Bottoms Up!

The Funny Side Collection

Wolfgang Amadeus Mozart (1756 – 1791) was a child prodigy who maintained a juvenile sense of humor throughout his relatively short but incredibly prolific and talented life. Some of his musical notes suggest the playing of a human wind instrument. He was obsessed with jokes about farts, farting, feces, analingus, and copraphilia.

James Gillray (1757-1815) was a noted English satirical cartoonist and printmaker. An etching he created entitled "Scientific Researches! —New Discoveries in PNEUMATICKS!" illustrates experiments with nitrous oxide (laughing gas) at the Royal Institution, where the subject of the inhalation of nitrous oxide releases a blast of gas as a fart.

A rare freshwater turtle in Australia can breathe through its cloaca / anus.

The Fart Side: Bottoms Up!

Utagawa Kuniyoshi (1797 - 1861) was a great master of the popular Japanese woodblock prints and painting. Amongst his many genres, he also created Japanese scroll paintings related to farting. These sell for very high prices, on the rare occasion when these prized works of fart art come up for auction.

Stoutshanks was a 19th century cartoonist and illustrator in England active from 1800 to 1830. He depicts the Duke of Wellington, who was then Prime Minister of England, astride a white swan propelled by farting.

Mr. Methane (Paul Oldfield) (1966-) is a British comedy stage performer who claims to be the world's only flatulist, a professional farter.

Ruminant livestock such as cattle release methane by burping.

The Fart Side: Bottoms Up!

Wilhelm Richard Wagner (1813 – 1883) was a German composer, theatre director, and conductor who was best known for his operas. He had chronic constipation that began in his twenties, and he would often refer to his lack of productivity, both as a digester and composer. He described the "birth of the tetralogy out of the low E flat of flatulence." He regularly complained of flatulence in both directions, referring to his frequent eructation in the same manner as his farts. He complained in intimate details of hemorrhoids, sluggishness of his 'unterleib', bloating, and flatulence. To assist his bowels, he regularly engaged in colonic irrigations, about which he wrote, that they "had become a new religion for me".

Lighting a cow manure patty is an unsafe way to demonstrate that they are flammable.

The Fart Side: Bottoms Up!

Joseph Pujol (1857 – 1945) was a stage performer from 1887 to 1914, and first performed on the Moulin Rouge stage in Paris in 1892. He had the ability to inhale air into his colon through his anus, and expel it at will. With the stage name Le Pétomane, French for the fart maniac, he was also affectionately known as 'the fartiste'. He would perform musical themes on his colonic 'wind instrument'.

The most common source of methane, comprising over twenty-five percent of the amount found in the atmosphere, is from termite farts.

Salvador Domingo Felipe Jacinto Dalí i Domènechl (1904 – 1989) was an eccentric and prominent Spanish surrealist painter born in the Catalonia region of Spain. He openly discussed his lifelong fascination and obsession with intestinal gas and farts.

The Fart Side: Bottoms Up!

Farts have been in movies from the very beginning, you just did not know it because they were silent films. It was said that Rudolph Valentino, the suave leading man of many romantic silent films, was notorious for his extensive and pungent farting on the film stage.

The presence of cinematic farts has been out of the bag for a long time, especially since the classic fart marathon of Mel Brook's *Blazing Saddles*. The character he plays, Governor Pétomane is named in honor of the famous Frenchman, Joseph Pujol, who brought farting to the heights of the entertainment world on Paris' famous Moulin Rouge under his stage name of Le Pétomane.

Over seventy percent of the free oxygen in the earth atmosphere is generated by marine Cyanobacteria and green algae.

The Fart Side: Bottoms Up!

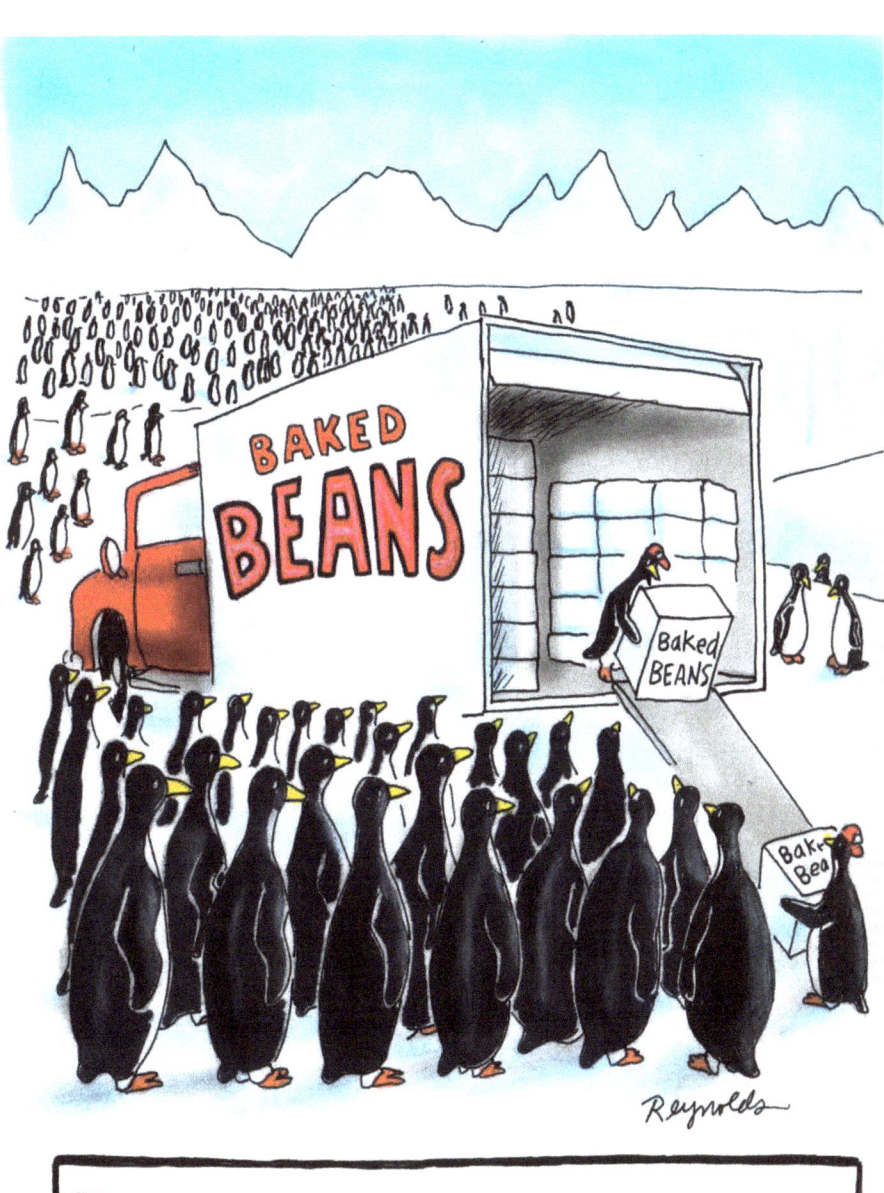

The well-known phenomenon of horse farts has been exploited on television, with an episode of the comedy series *Seinfeld* entitled *The Rye*. Cramer feeds the horse pulling a hansom carriage in Central Park in New York City a meal that makes the horse extremely flatulent, to great comedic effect

The Lion King was a very successful award winning animated motion picture, and Broadway musical, produced by Walt Disney Studios. The song *Hakuna Matata* has the meerkat Timor leading, and the warthog Pumbaa as an ever-farting sidekick. Pumbaa nearly gets the word fart into the lyrics, until warned by Timor not to say the word in front of the children.

The main reason a dead body floats is because of the gas that continues to be produced in the intestinal tract even after death.

The Fart Side: Bottoms Up!

An equine fart theme took place in a Super Bowl advertisement for Budweiser beer. A man and a young woman are in a romantic horse drawn carriage. He presents her with a lit candle and reaches down to pull up some bottles of Budweiser beer. As he is bending over and out of the way getting the beer, the horse's tail lifts. The horse farts and the candle explodes in a ball of flame obscuring the young woman's facial features. When the man sits back upright, oblivious to what happened, he smells smoke and asks if she smells a barbeque.

Charles de Gaulle (1890 – 1970) French general, statesman, and gourmand, blamed his farts on dishes prepared from offal.

Methane is twenty times as potent a greenhouse gas as carbon dioxide.

The Fart Side: Bottoms Up!

The average person swallows two thousand times per day, and each swallow includes five milliliters (one teaspoon) of air. The ten liters of air swallowed every day is seventy- eight percent nitrogen, which since it is not well absorbed, must be released as a burp or as a fart.

The musk scent gland of deer is a very expensive ingredient frequently used in perfumes. Although the word musk means testicle in the Sanskrit language, it is a misnomer and is only found in the female of the species.

Toilet paper was first used in ancient China. Hardwood pulp was often used in early toilet paper, and the risk of a wood splinter after wiping was a real concern.

Herring and other fish communicate by releasing gas bubbles underwater.

The Fart Side: Bottoms Up!

The use of human feces as a fertilizer, known as night soil, is common in many parts of the world.

Oxygen (Greek for acid producer) was given its name in error, it is hydrogen not oxygen that is a requirement for acid production.

One gram (one thirtieth of an ounce) of diarrhea from a child with rotavirus contains enough infectious virus particles to infect every human on earth, and ten thousand additional planets that had an equivalent human population.

Petrified dinosaur poop, called a coprolite or coprolith, is a valuable find prized by paleontologists.

The dung beetle which collects animal droppings was considered sacred in Ancient Egypt.

The Fart Side: Bottoms Up!

The intestinal tract has pacemaker cells, like those of the heart.

The intestinal tract has a complex nervous system that allows communication between the brain, gut, microbiome, and diet.

Gastroesophageal reflux can cause earaches, asthma, sinusitis, sleep disorder, cough, ear infection, laryngitis, heartburn, and a higher risk of esophageal cancer.

The average length of the human small intestine is twenty-three feet (seven meters).

The term for heartburn is pyrosis.

About twenty percent of bioactive metabolites circulating in human blood originates from microbes living within the gut.

The Fart Side: Bottoms Up!

There appears to be a correlation between the gut microbiome and many disorders, including autism, depression, anxiety, obsessive compulsive disorder, obesity, arthritis, cardiovascular disease, inflammatory bowel disease, irritable bowel syndrome, leaky gut syndrome, Parkinson Disease, and Alzheimer Disease.

The primary physiologic stimulus for breathing is the buildup of the level of carbon dioxide in the blood, not the level of oxygen.

The detection of a fart requires that the odorant molecules that arose in the intestinal tract, and was released as a fart, had to travel all the way to your nose, and have direct contact direct with the cilia receptors of your olfactory nerve cell.

The Fart Side: Bottoms Up!

Produced in salivary glands, human saliva is 99.5% water, but it contains many important substances, including electrolytes, mucus, antibacterial compounds and various enzymes.

Modifications of saliva in other animals includes the venom of snakes, and the thread of some spiders and caterpillars. The swift bird uses its gummy saliva to build its bird nest, which is used in the Chinese delicacy of bird nest soup.

Salivary lipase allows fat digestion to take place even in conditions where the lipase from the pancreas is absent.

Amylase in saliva begins the digestive process of carbohydrates, breaking complex starches into simple sugars. Eating a potato chip, the enzymes release sugars from starch, giving a sweet taste promptly with chewing.

The Fart Side: Bottoms Up!

"The coffee was bound to be good here. After all, 'Fine Café' is an anagram for 'caffeine'."

Technically the digestive tract isn't internal or *inside* the body, it is external or *outside*. It is a hollow canal that is open to the external environment, all the way from the mouth to the anus.

The digestive system is the origin of more cancers, and is responsible for more cancer deaths each year, than any other organ system in the body.

Laundry detergents are designed like digestive juices, they often contain several different classes of enzymes, including proteases to digest proteins, amylases to digest carbohydrates, and lipases to digest fats.

The mouth, teeth, tongue, and salivary glands chew food, which is called a bolus when swallowed. When the partly digested material leaves the stomach, it is called chime.

The Fart Side: Bottoms Up!

Some animals, including seahorses, lungfishes and platypuses, have no stomach. Their food goes from the esophagus straight to the intestines.

Each year, more than 270,000 Americans develop a cancer of the gastrointestinal tract, including cancers of the esophagus, stomach, colon and rectum. About half of these cancers result in death.

Colorectal cancer kills more than 50,000 people in the U.S. each year, more than any other cancer except lung cancer.

An endoscope is an instrument used to examine organs and cavities inside the body.

Some gallstones, made from calcium and extra fatty cholesterols, can be dissolved with bile acid supplements.

The Fart Side: Bottoms Up!

An adult esophagus ranges from ten to fourteen inches in length, and one inch in diameter.

The gallbladder stores the bile secreted by the liver, and releases it into the duodenum of the small intestine when food rich in cholesterol or other lipids is ingested.

The bile secreted by the gall bladder emulsifies fat molecules so that fat digestive enzymes, like lipase, can carry out their breakdown and digestion effectively.

The large intestine is approximately five feet (1.5 meters) long, and three inches (7.5 centimeters) in diameter.

Removing the gallbladder does not interfere significantly with fat metabolism, as the bile is directly secreted to the intestine.

The Fart Side: Bottoms Up!

Rapid weight loss is a risk factor for the development of gallstones.

Swallowing is a complex procedure in which the bolus is moved into the pharynx. The larynx (vocal cords/voice-box) and trachea (windpipe) is protected by closure of the epiglottis. The upper esophageal sphincter is relaxed to accept the bolus. The bolus is then moved through the esophagus, through coordinated muscle movements known as peristalsis.

The esophagus is bound on each end by a sphincter muscle, which is responsible for opening to allow the bolus to pass through. Heartburn can occur when the lower sphincter fails to close completely, or relaxes at the wrong time, allowing stomach acid to travel upward with regurgitation or reflux, and irritate the tissue in the esophagus and throat.

The Fart Side: Bottoms Up!

The gallbladder empties bile, a yellowish and greenish fluid from the liver, into the duodenum when chyme enters that portion of the intestine. Although bile does not contain enzymes, it does have bile salts that help dissolve fats.

The gallbladder concentrates the bile acid content of the bile tenfold.

The duodenum is one-foot-long, and is named for the Greek description of 'two hands in size'. It receives the chyme leaving the stomach at the pyloric valve, and contains the entry points for the addition of pancreatic enzymes and sodium bicarbonate from the pancreatic duct, and bile from the liver and gallbladder from the common bile duct. They enter together through the anatomical Sphincter of Oddi, at the Ampulla of Vater.

The Fart Side: Bottoms Up!

Fly Commercials

Digested carbohydrates, fats, proteins, and most of the vitamins, minerals, and iron in food are absorbed in the jejunum, which is about four feet (1.2 meters) long. Aiding this absorption are up to five million tiny finger-like projections called *villi,* which greatly increase the surface area of the small intestine, thus accelerating the rate at which nutrients are absorbed into the bloodstream.

The remainder of the small intestine is taken up by the ileum, which is smaller in diameter, and has thinner walls than the jejunum. It is the final site for absorption of some vitamins, bile acids, and other nutrients, which enter the circulatory system in plasma, a watery liquid in which red blood cells also are suspended.

The main function of the colon is to remove and conserves water.

The Fart Side: Bottoms Up!

The large intestine removes and conserves water from the remaining fiber and waste material transiting the colon. In addition, the trillions of microbes in the gut microbiome produce certain B vitamins and vitamin K, which are absorbed into the bloodstream along with the water. They also produce short chain fatty acids which serve as an energy source for colonic cells.

The movement of food through the entire length of the digestive tract takes up to thirty hours, with most that time being taken up by activity in the colon. Food generally spends about three to five hours in the stomach, another four to five hours in the small intestine, and between five and twenty-four hours in the large intestine. The transit time is a function of diet: for a vegetarian who eats a great deal of fiber, it will be shorter.

The Fart Side: Bottoms Up!

The gas production that results from eating beans can be dramatically reduced by allowing them to sprout before cooking and eating. The beans have complex sugars such as raffinose, stachyose, and verbascose that cannot be digested by humans, and end up being fermented by the gut microbes producing gas. They are broken down into absorbable simple sugars by the enzyme alpha-galactosidase which is released by the plant upon with sprouting.

Human feces are given many names, including number two, bowel movement (B.M.), excrement, poop, shit, dung, doo, crap, dump, and hundreds of other euphemisms.

The average person excretes about seven pounds (3.2 kg) of feces per day, equal to a little more than one ton per year.

The Fart Side: Bottoms Up!

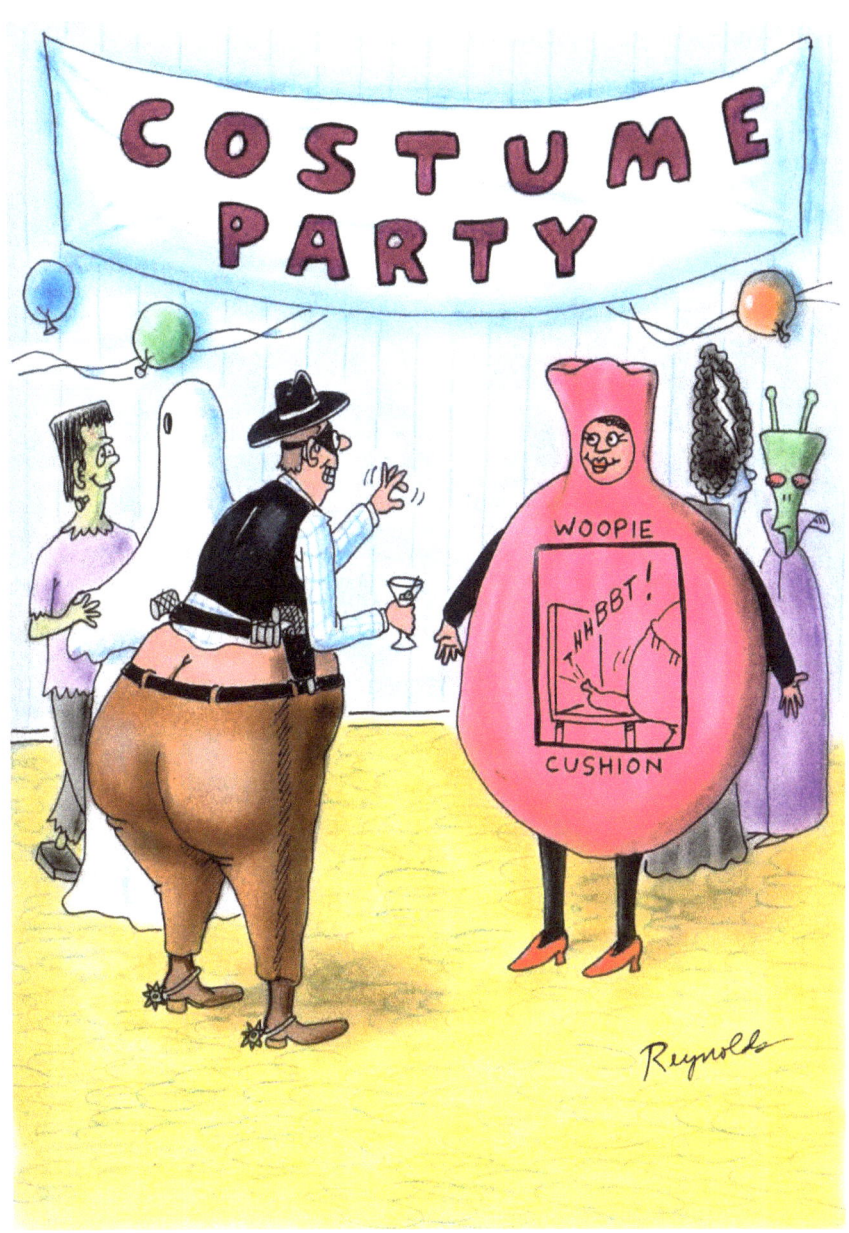

The Funny Side Collection

Dan Reynolds
Joseph Weiss, MD

Dan Reynolds
Joseph Weiss, MD

Dan Reynolds
Joseph Weiss, MD

Dan Reynolds
Joseph Weiss, MD

Available in 5"x7" (96 pages) Pocket Rocket! & 6"x9" (122 pages) Expanded Full Blast! print/e-book edition

www.thefunnysidecollection.com

The Fart Side: Bottoms Up!

Dan Reynolds

Dan Reynolds began drawing cartoons in December of 1989. He draws and eats left-handed. He plays ping pong and pool left-handed. He throws, kicks and bats right-handed. Like a box of chocolates, you never know what you're going to get, but you will like most of them and they'll keep you coming back. Unlike chocolates, REYNOLDS UNWRAPPED cartoons are not fattening.

The Funny Side Collection

Dan's cartoons are seen by millions of readers across the U.S., Canada, and points beyond all the way down under in Australia. His work is seen in every issue of Reader's Digest (where he is known for his cow, pig, and chicken cartoons).

His cartoons have appeared on HBO's The Sopranos, the cover of a National Lampoon cartoon book collection, and on greeting cards all throughout the United States. His work also appears in many other places as well.

Sign-up for Dan's daily REYNOLDS UNWRAPPED e-mail cartoon for only $12 for a whole year. E-mail Dan at reynoldsunwrapped@gmail.com for details. Dan's website is:
www.reynoldsunwrapped.weebly.com

The Fart Side series and other items are available at:
   www.thefunnysidecollection.com

The Fart Side: Bottoms Up!

Joseph Weiss, M.D.

GI Joe is Clinical Professor of Medicine in the Division of Gastroenterology at the University of California, San Diego. He is a Fellow of the American College of Physicians, Fellow of the American Gastroenterological Association, and a Senior Fellow of the American College of Gastroenterology.

Dr. Weiss is the author of several dozen books on health available at:
www.smartaskbooks.com

He is an accomplished professional speaker and humorist, having given over three thousand invited presentations internationally at universities, international conventions, conferences, corporations, resorts, and special events.

The Fart Side series and other items are available at:
www.thefunnysidecollection.com

"Dr. Joseph Weiss' books provide an informative and entertaining approach to sharing insights about our digestive system and wellbeing." **Deepak Chopra, MD**

"Joseph Weiss, M.D. has a gift for books that are uniquely informative and entertaining. **Jack Canfield** Coauthor of the Chicken Soup for the Soul® series

The Fart Side: Bottoms Up!

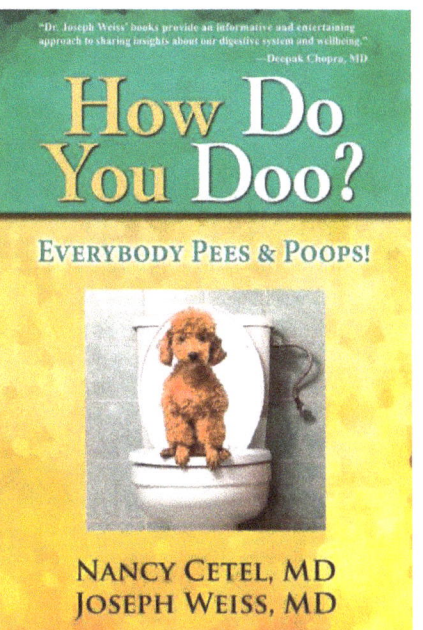

www.smartaskbooks.com

The Funny Side Collection

www.smartaskbooks.com

www.ingramcontent.com/pod-product-compliance
Lightning Source LLC
Chambersburg PA
CBHW041958080526
44588CB00021B/2785